💕 THIS BOOK IS DEDICATED TO 💕

ALL THE PEDIATRIC DENTISTS, GENERAL DENTISTS, AND DENTAL HYGIENISTS WHOSE TENDER LOVING CARE PREVENTS FEAR AND ANXIETY AMONGST THEIR TINY, TRUSTING PATIENTS

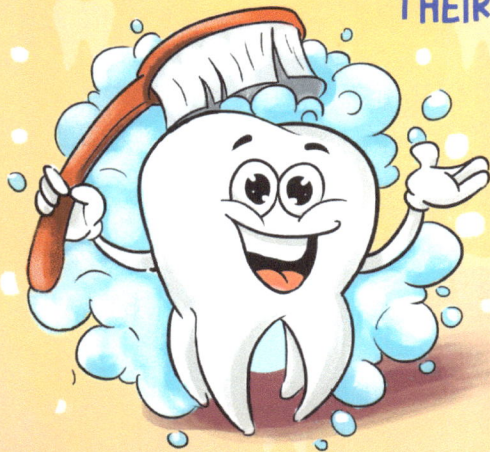

Follow the (NOT) Scary Series a

www.tanaholmes.com

🐦 @TanaHolmesAuthr

📷 tanaholmesauthor

f TanaHolmesAuthor

ISBN: 978-1-7364387-3-2 Hardcover/978-1-7364387-4-9 Paperback
Text and illustrations copyright © 2022 by Tana Holmes Girasol Publishing, LLC

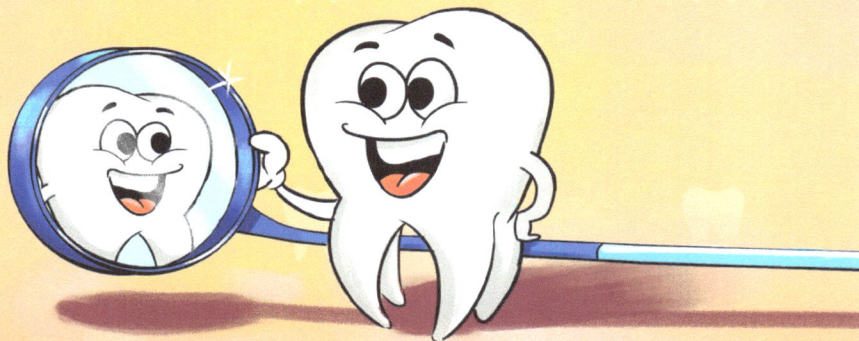

When babies are born, you can't see their teeth.
They're in there, just hidden underneath.

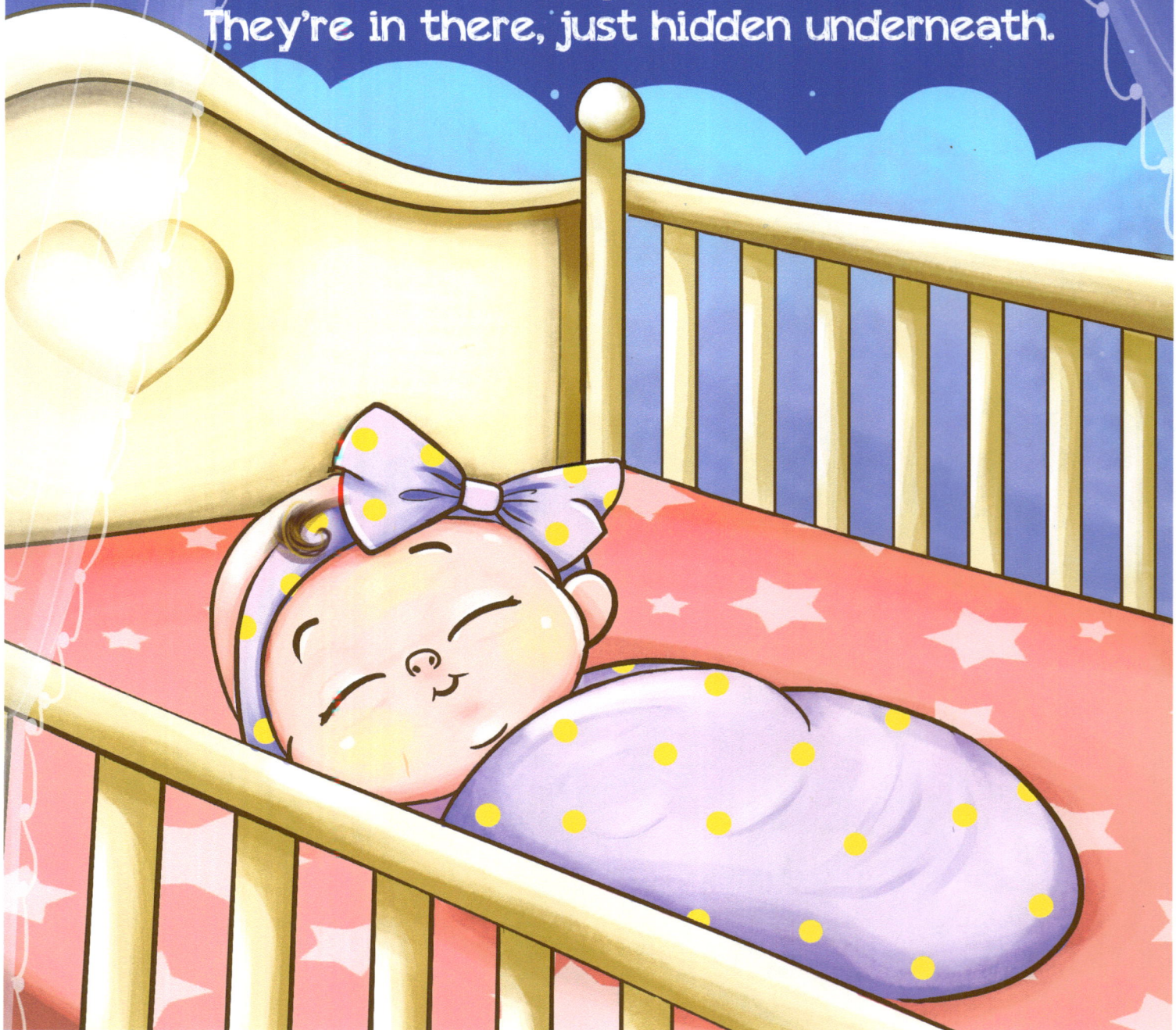

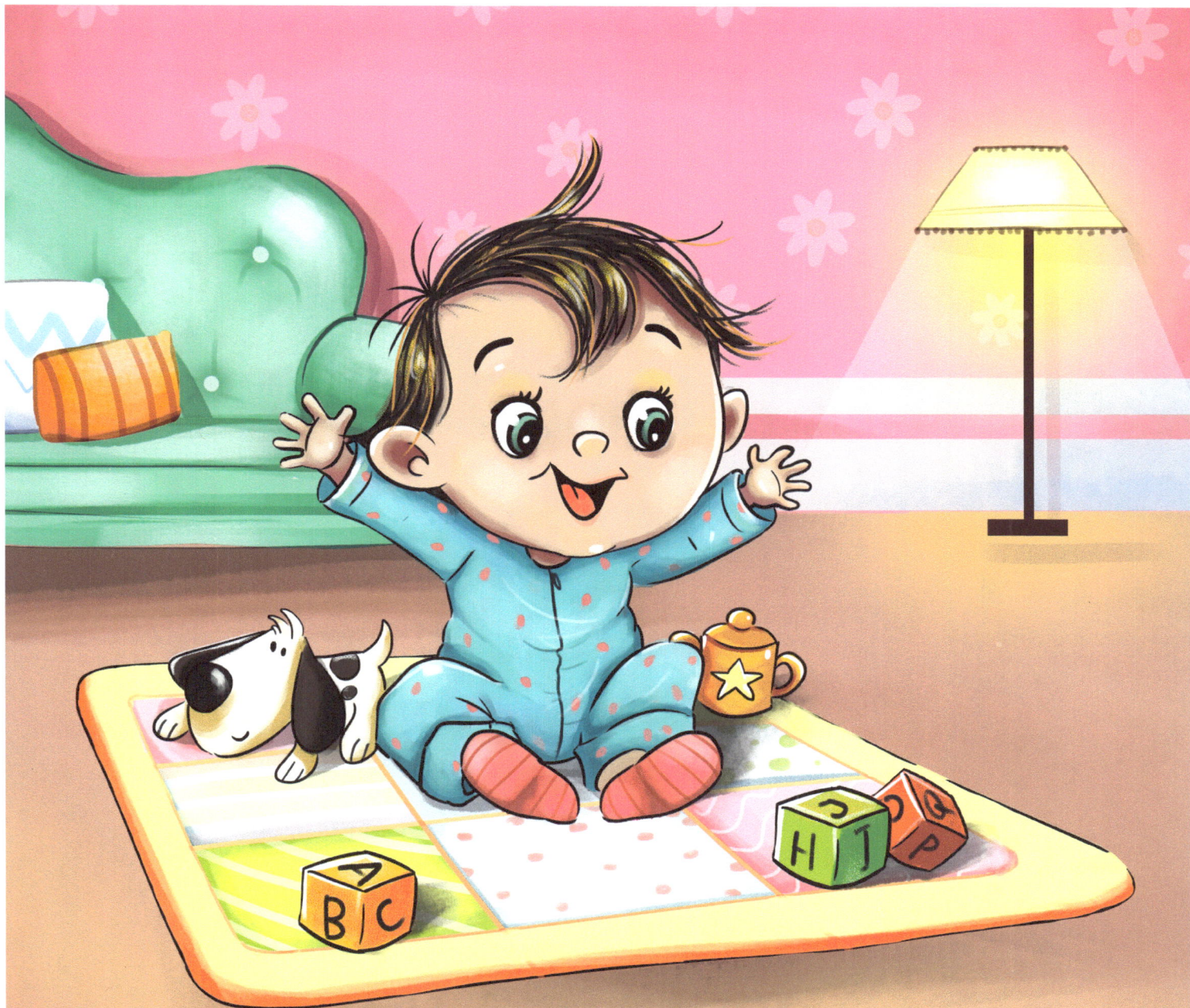

One by one your baby teeth pop out
until they form a pretty smile for everyone to check out!

When you grow a bit more, your "baby teeth" start to wiggle.
Then one will fall out, and the rest start to jiggle!

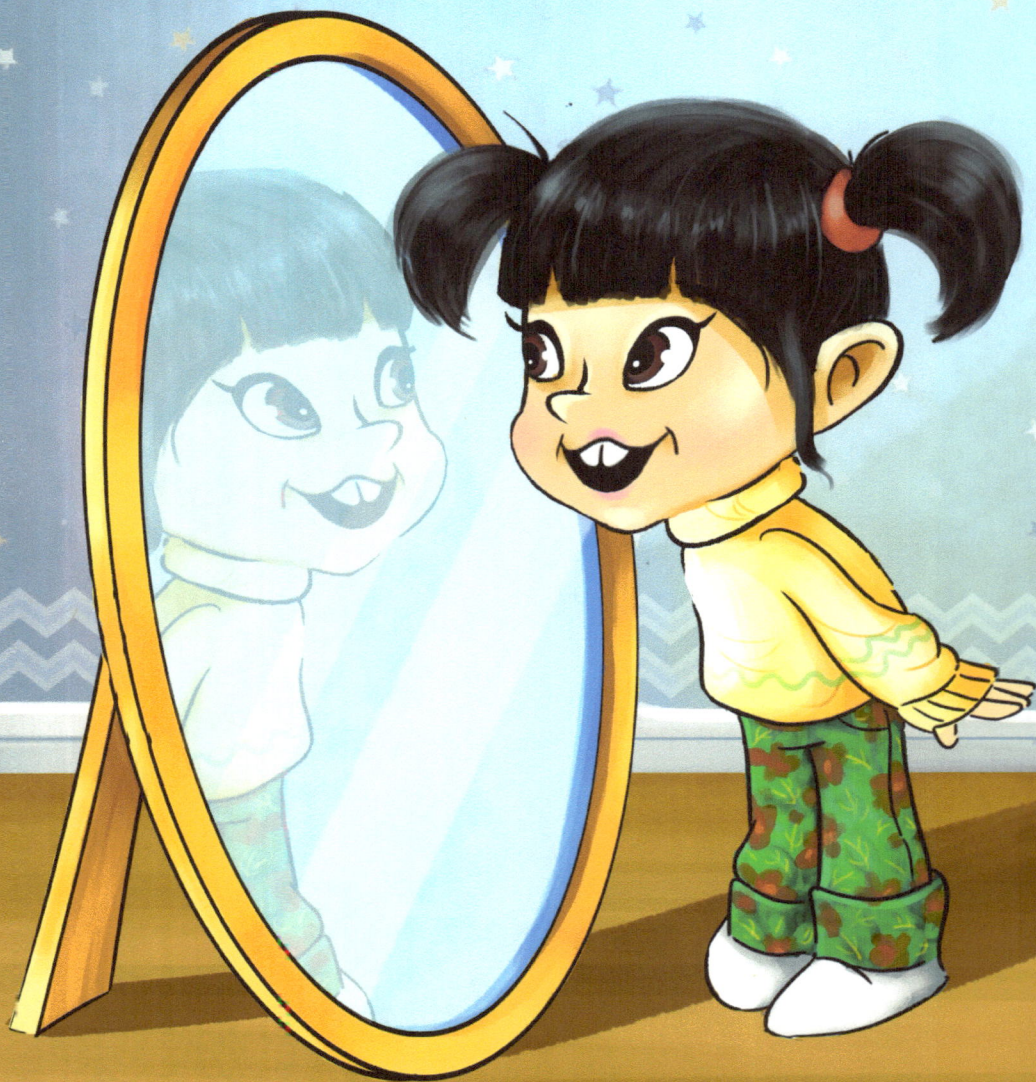

But it's okay, don't be sad.
You'll soon have grown-up teeth like your mom and dad.

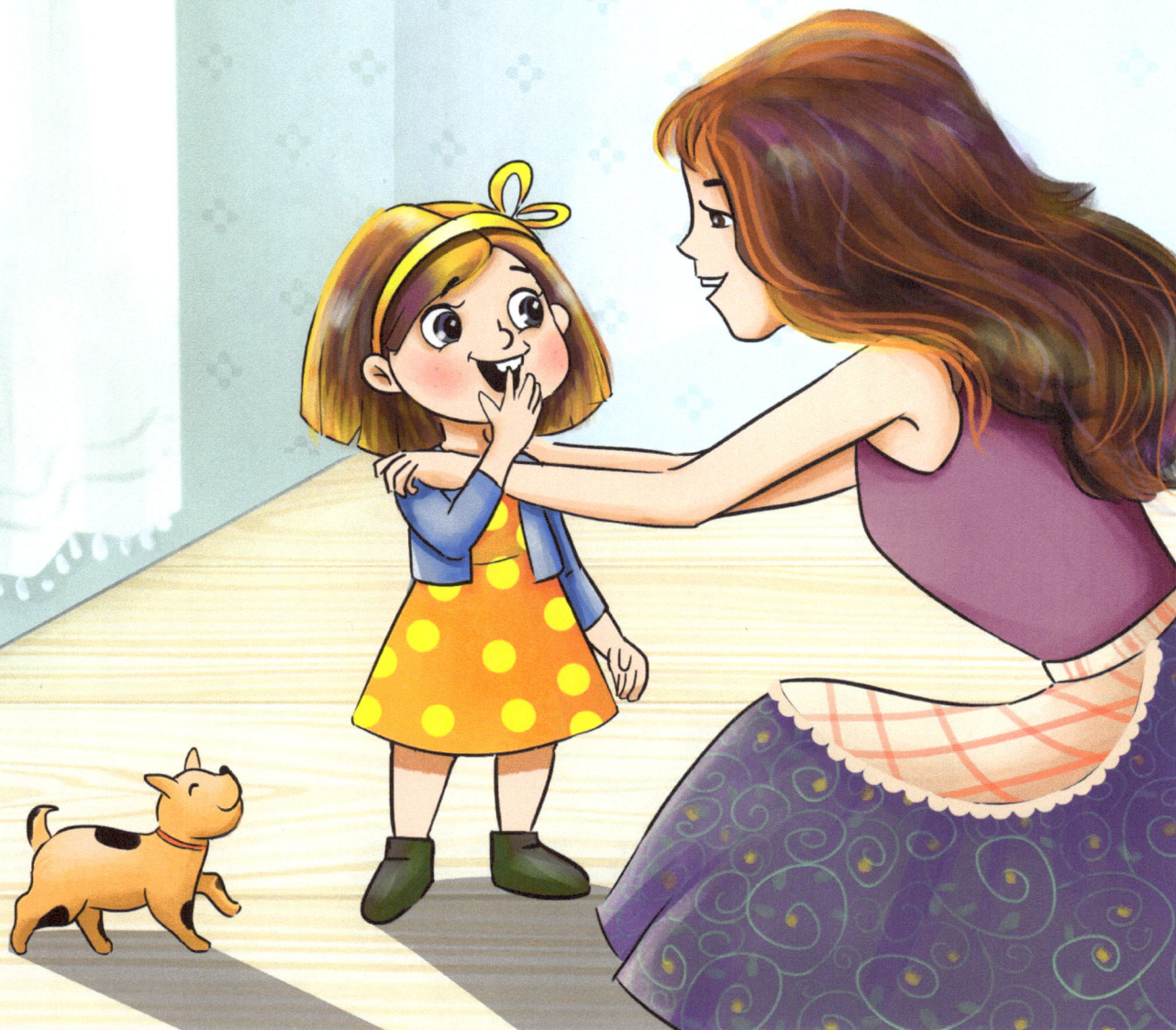

Your new teeth are treasures that need gentle care.
But they are under attack, so pull up a chair.
Let's learn what to do so you won't be scared.

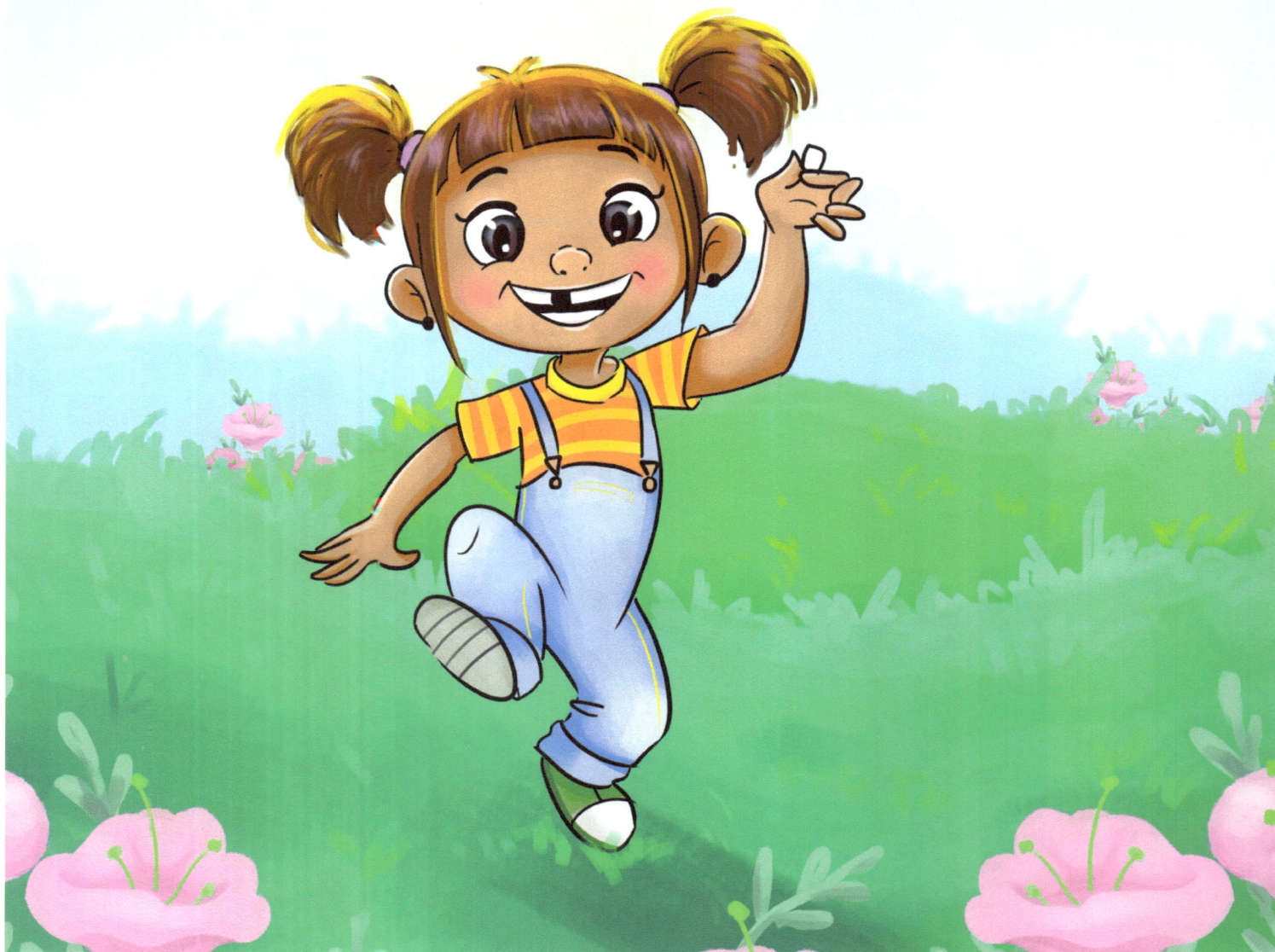

When you chew sticky food, your teeth are a trap.
That food stays in there for the Sugar Bugs to snack!
They chew a hole in the tooth's shiny white part.
They dig and dig once they get a little start.

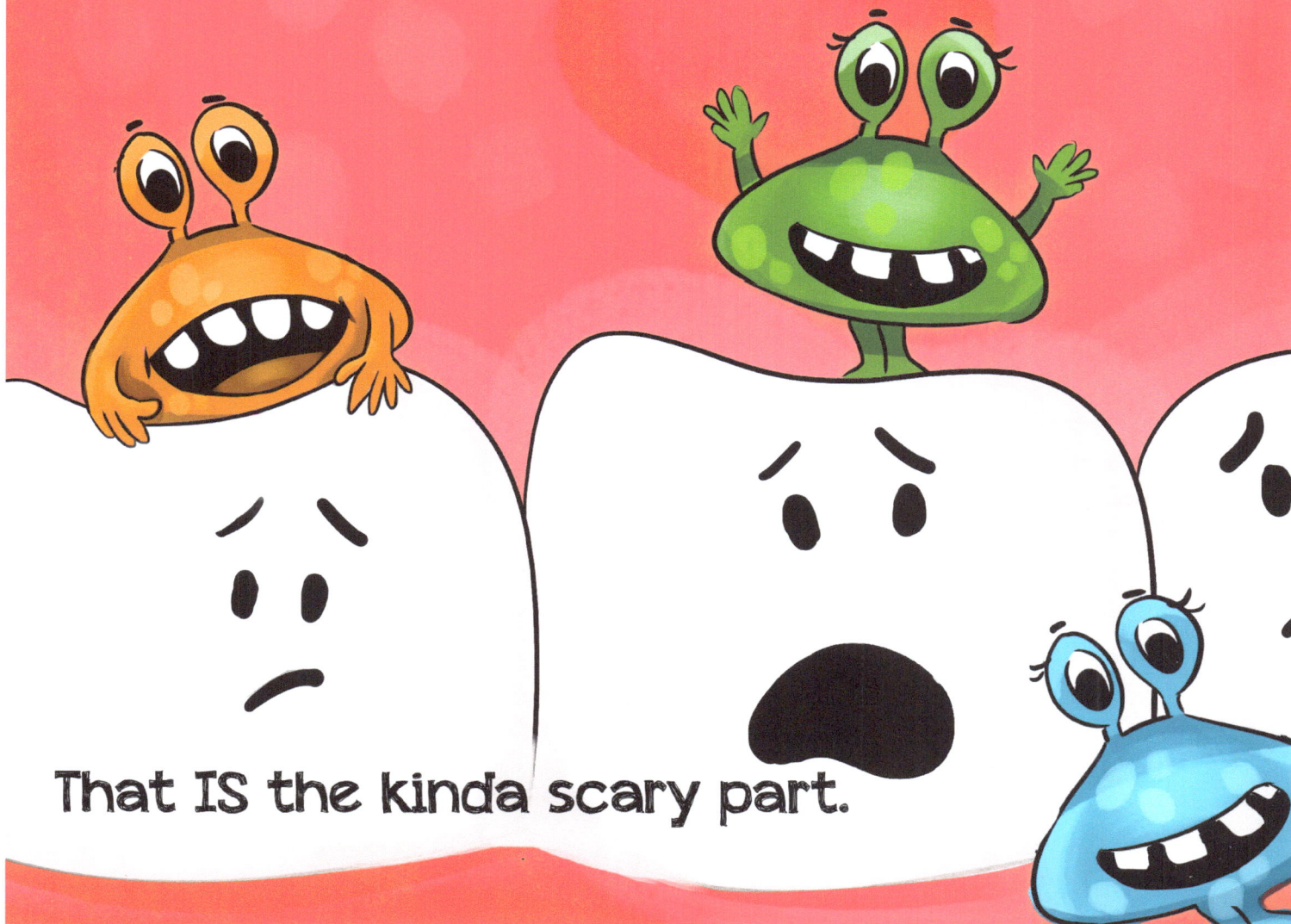

That IS the kinda scary part.

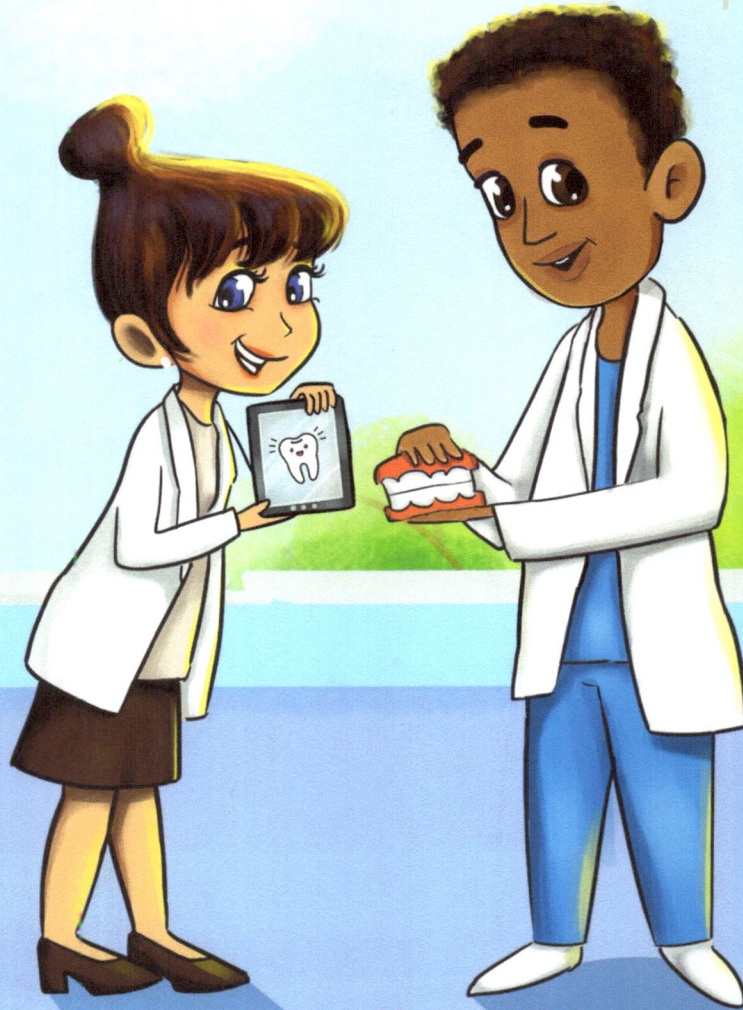

Did you know there are neighborhood friends
that help keep the SUGAR BUGS away?
They are Dentists and Dental Hygienists.

And they're NOT a bit SCARY!
Hip-hip-hooray!

Our dental friends work in an Office or Clinic.

They have comfy chairs, flashing lights, and even TVs.
Others have aquariums and playrooms to put you at ease.

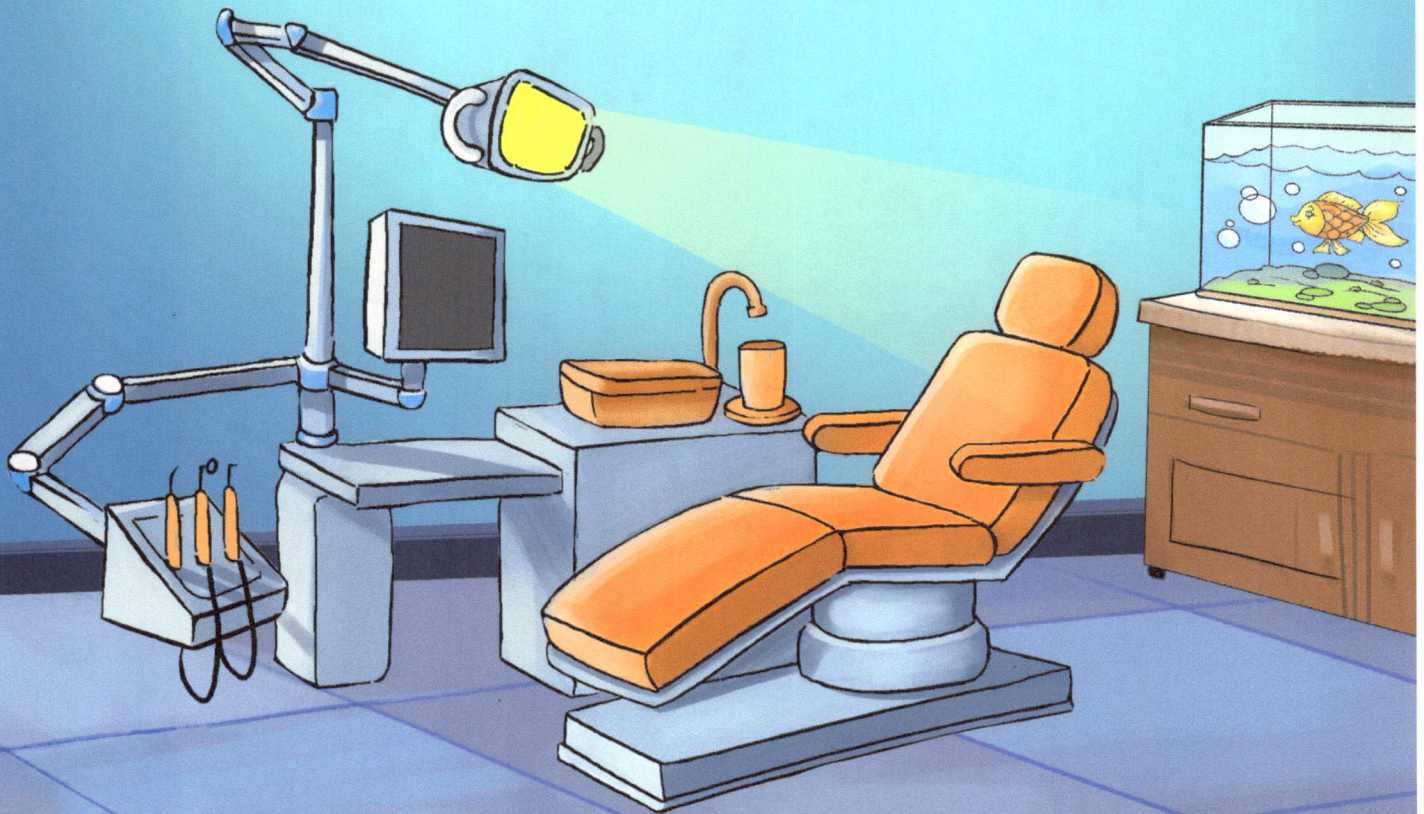

Definitely **NOT SCARY** !

Cool Shades

The chair is soft and leans all the way back.
The dentist is ready to keep you snug and relaxed.
You'll even get sunglasses to guard your eyes.
Before you go home, you'll get a fun prize!

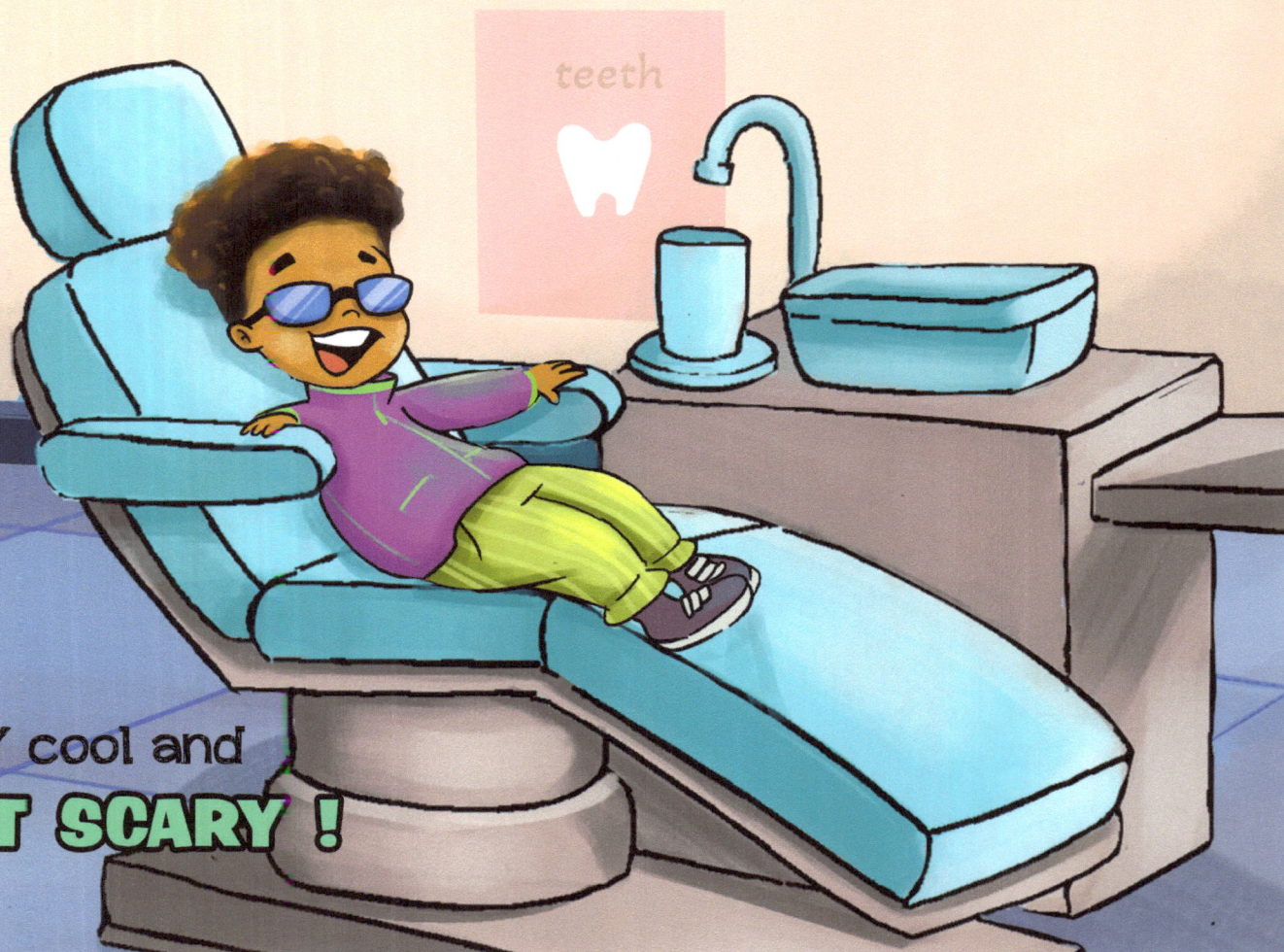

teeth

VERY cool and
NOT SCARY !

The Tooth Counter and Tiny Mirror

How many shiny white teeth live in your pretty pink gums?
You start with 20 baby teeth, then 32 when the time comes!
The tooth counter and mirror help with the count.
One, two, three, four...just the right amount.

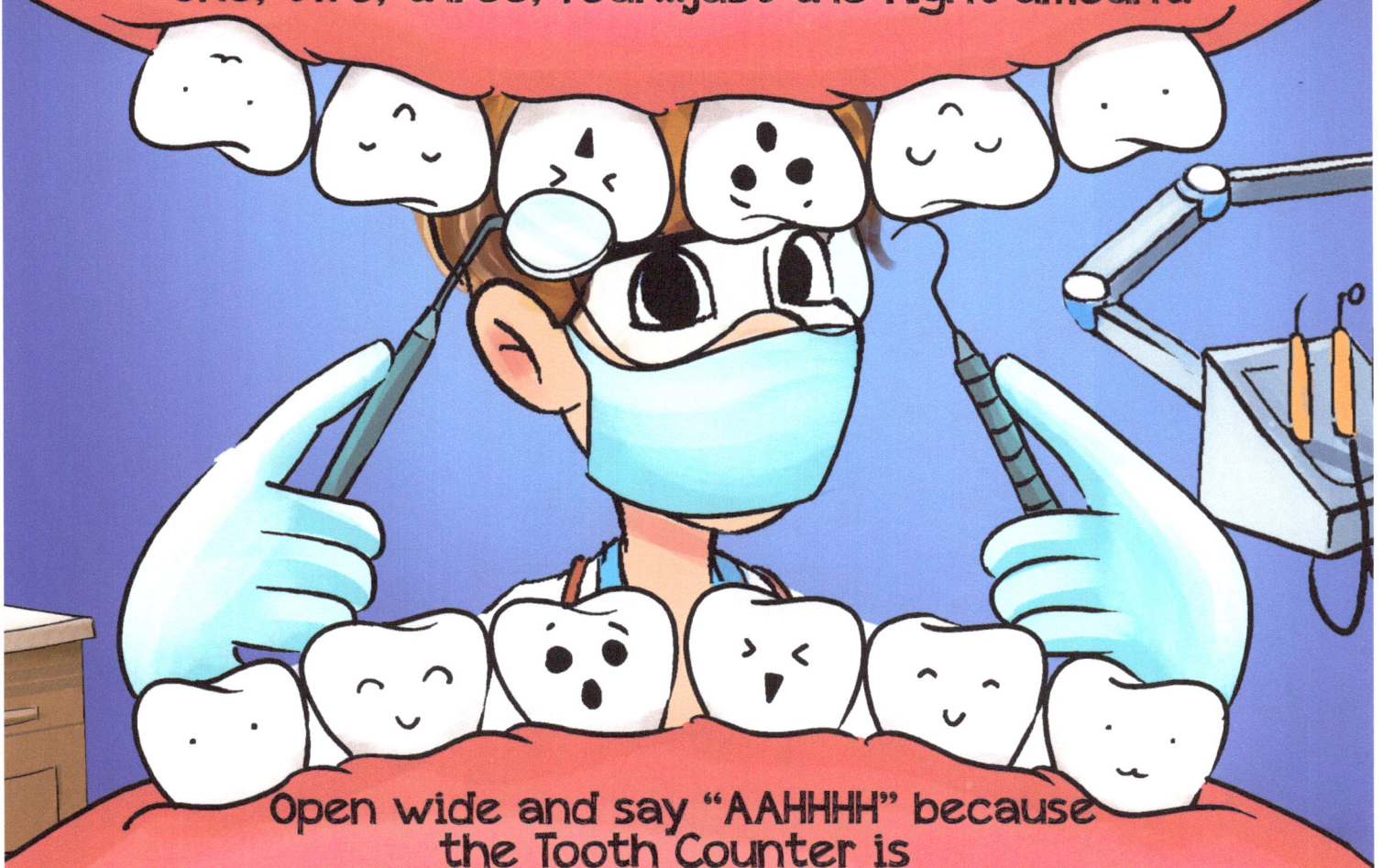

Open wide and say "AAHHHH" because
the Tooth Counter is

NOT SCARY!

Picture Time !

X-Rays are just pictures of your teeth.
They look like this, can you see the roots underneath?

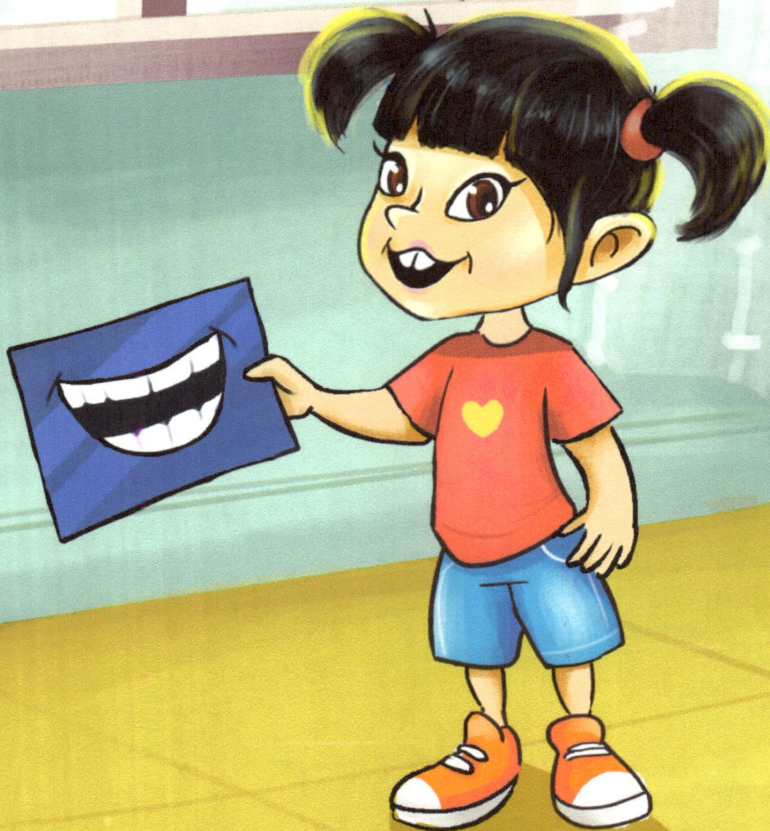

It doesn't hurt at all, and it's...
NOT SCARY!

The Water Squirter and Mr. Thirsty

Everyone takes a bath, or at least they oughta.
Water Squirter washes your teeth
and Mr. Thirsty straw sucks up the water.

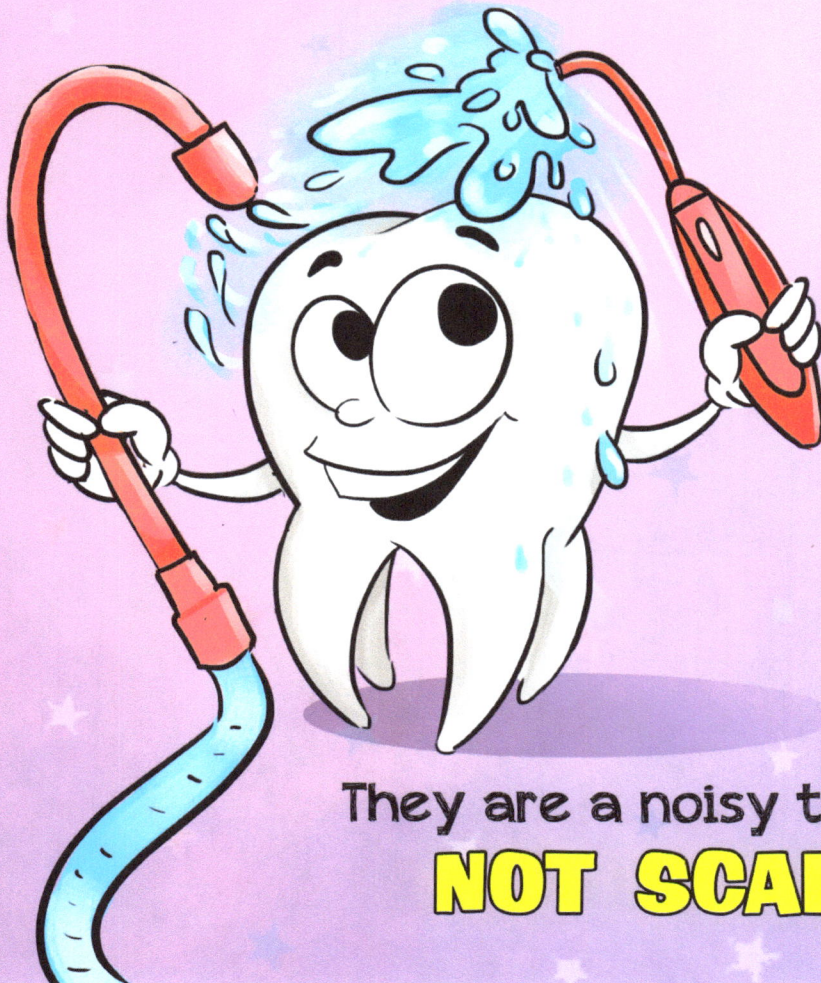

They are a noisy team. but
NOT SCARY!

The Teeth Tickler

The hygienist has a spinning tooth tickler
that shines up your teeth, it couldn't be simpler!
A few minutes of polishing that tastes like berry...

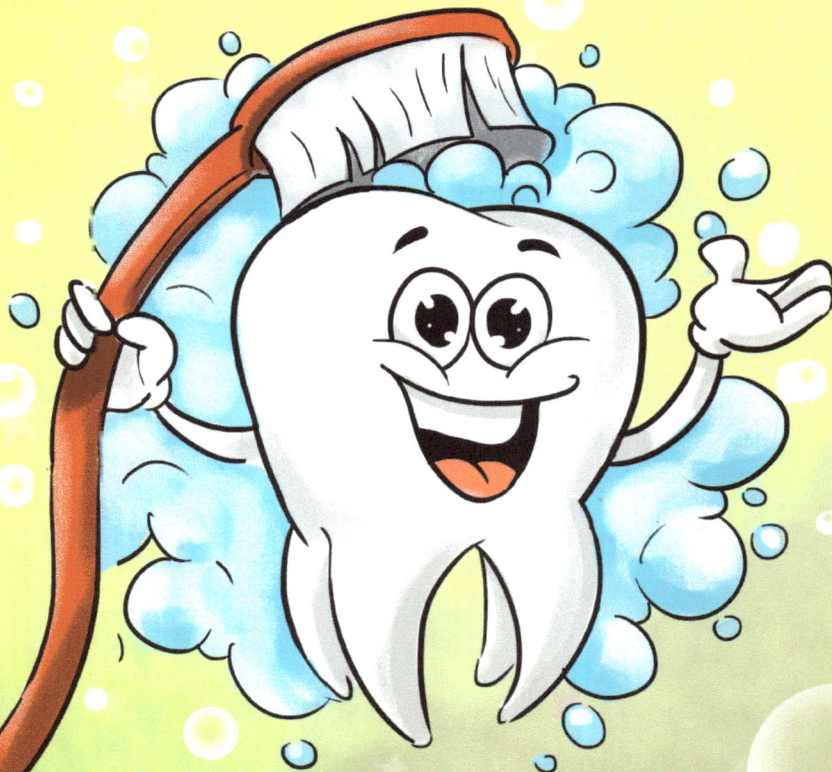

Let's say it together,
NOT SCARY!

Cavities

The tooth hole the Sugar Bugs chew is a cavity.
If you get one, you must alert your family.
If it gets any bigger it will start to hurt,
so to the dentist you go- they're the cavity experts.

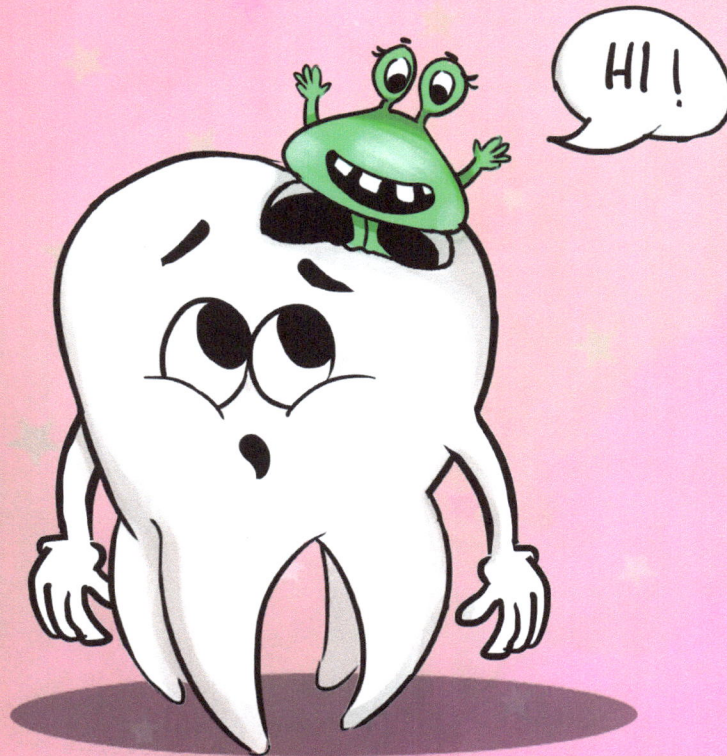

HI !

Sleepy Juice

"Sleepy Juice" goes next to your tooth in one little spot,
or is breathed through a mask like an astronaut.
It makes your tooth take a nap. Medicine in, repairs in a snap!

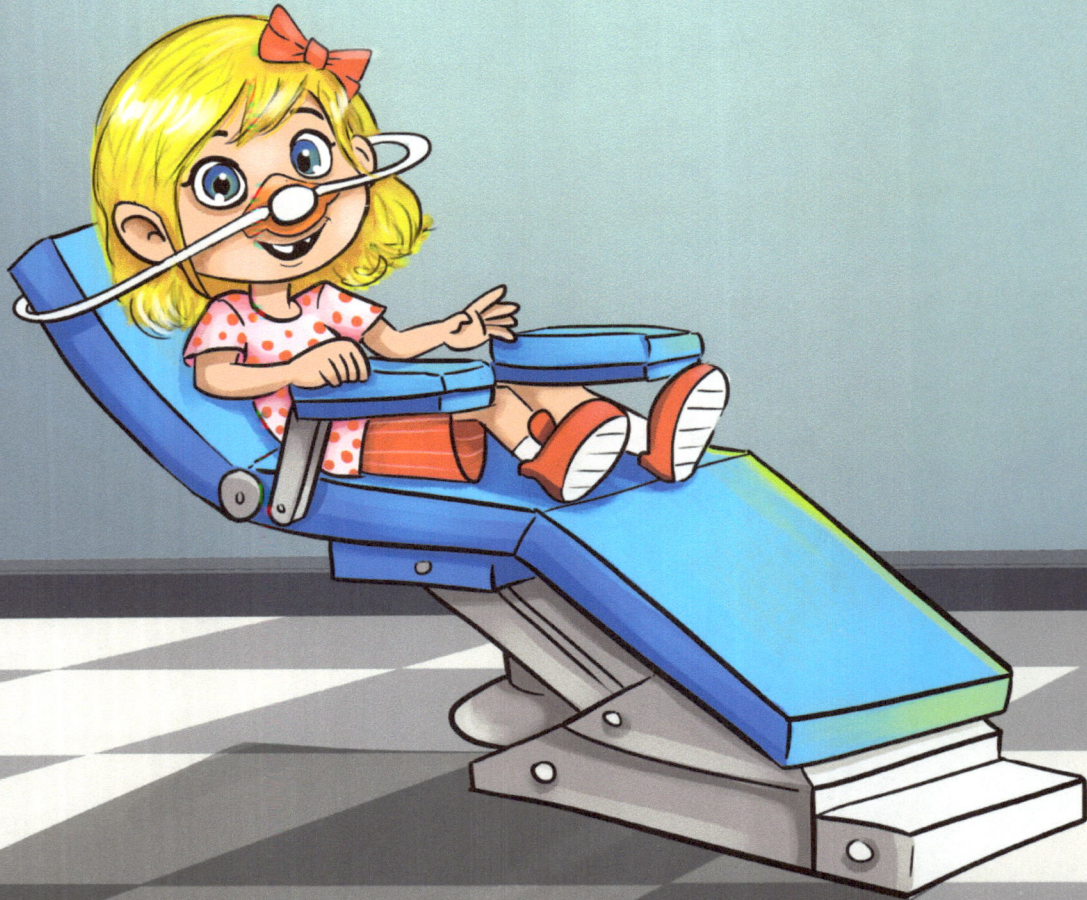

And it's **NOT SCARY!**

Mr. Bumpy

Now that your Sugar Bug tooth is asleep,
the dentist cleans the brown away in one big sweep.
A whistling brush called "Mr Bumpy" scrubs the yucky brown hole.
Then a wash by Water Squirter and Thirsty gets you to your goal.

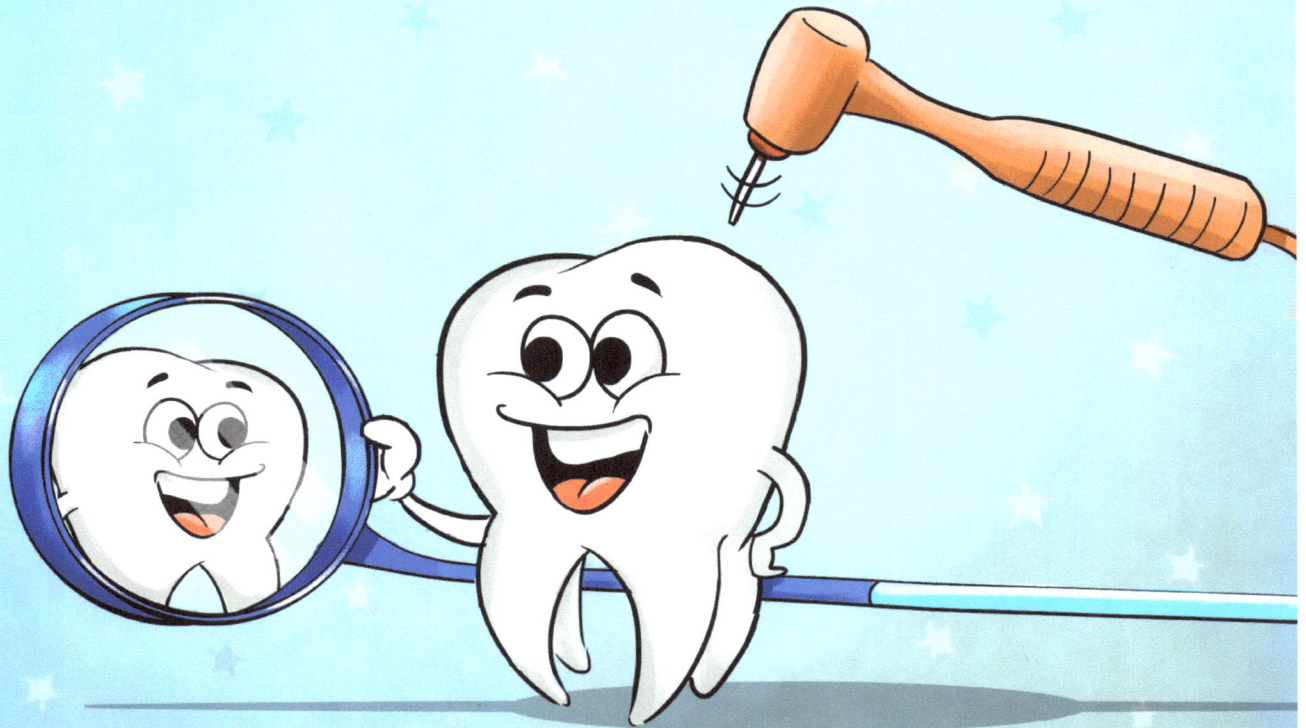

It sounds like a buzzing bee but it's

NOT SCARY!!

Filling

Next the dentist fills the hole
by putting in some white dough.
a light is shined to make the dough bind.

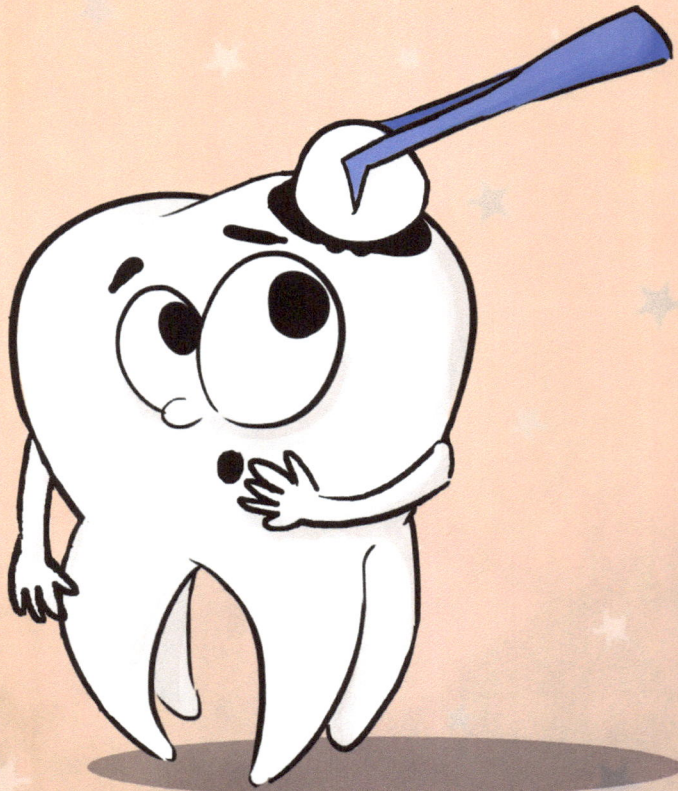

Then...

All Better!

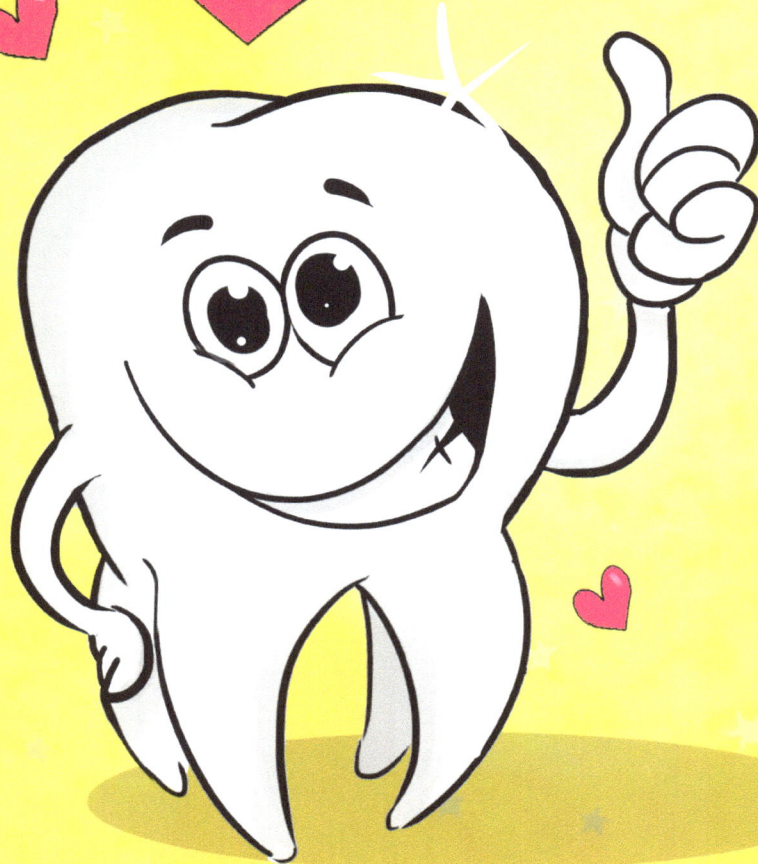

Now it's IMPORTANT to keep the Bugs from getting in again.
Here are some healthy ideas to put in your brain.

The Toothbrush

Choose your favorite color toothbrush and give it a name.
Brush little circles, play a song, make it a game!
Pick out a fun one with an elephant or superhero.
How many SUGAR BUGS now? Absolutely ZERO!

Toothbrushes are
NOT SCARY!

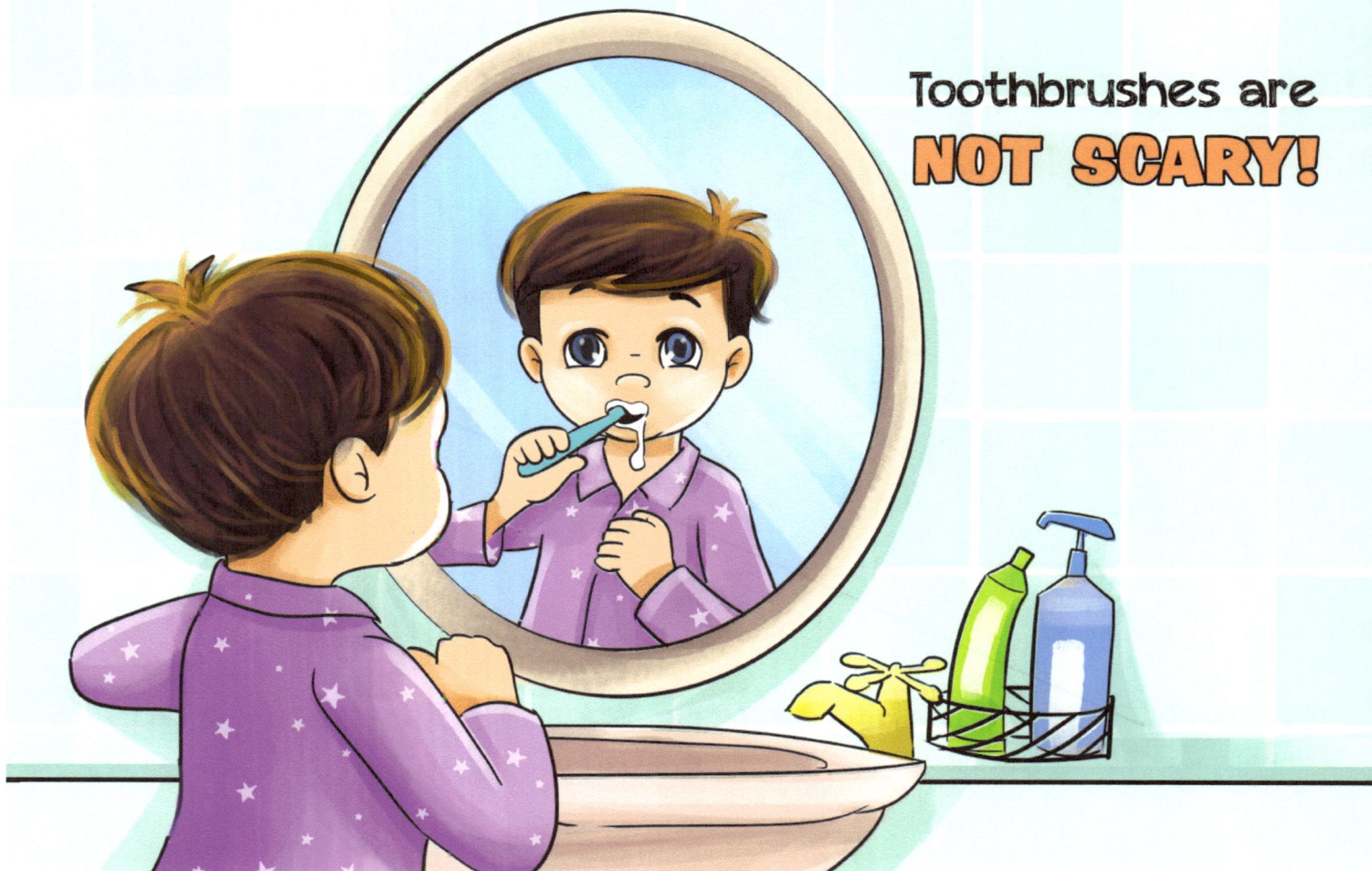

Dental Floss

Remember those spaces between your teeth?
"You-know-who" comes back to hide
if sticky food stays while you sleep
(Psst- "You-Know-Who" means the SUGAR BUGS!!)

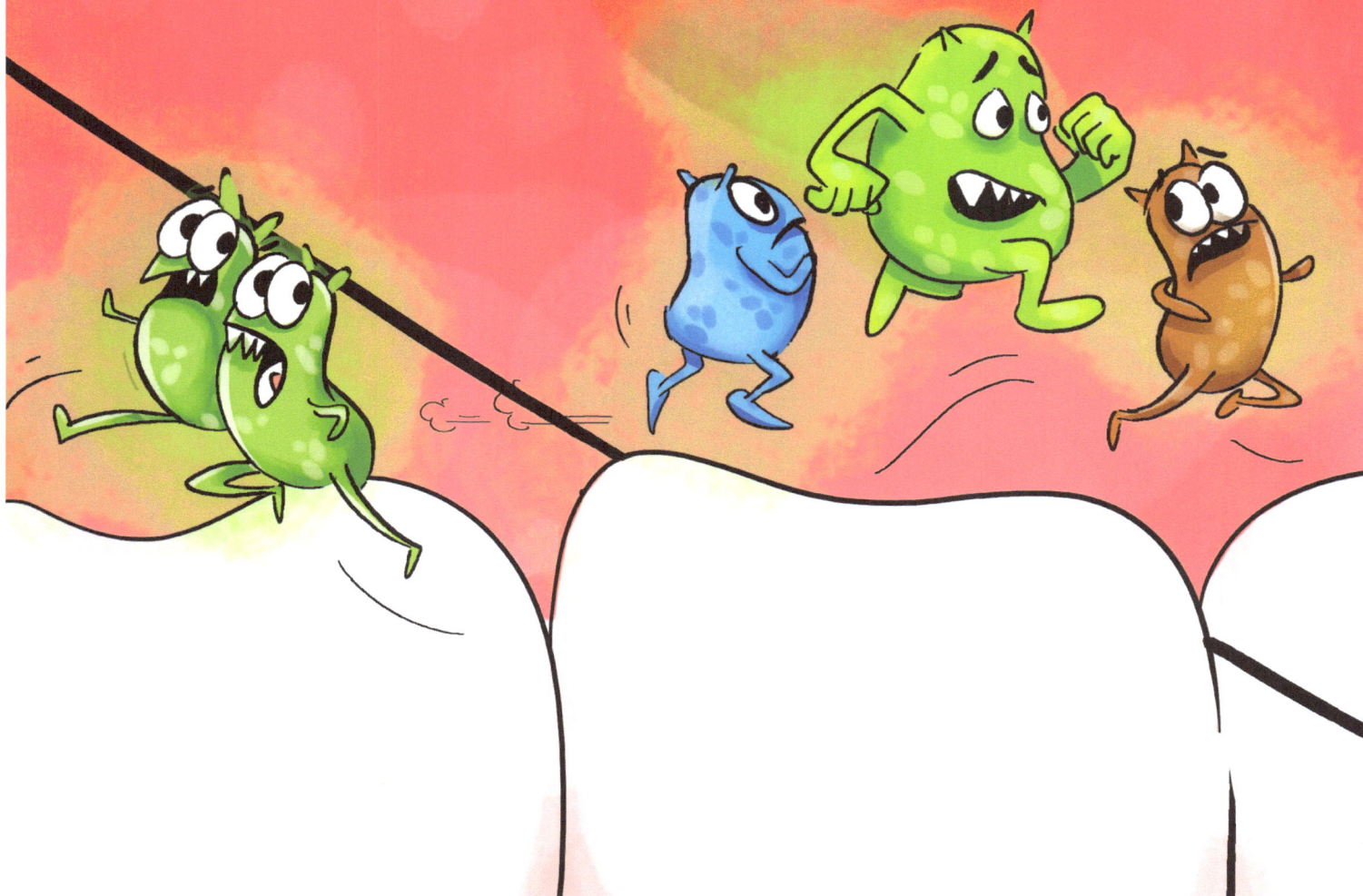

Your dentist, hygienist, or grown-ups at your home
can teach you how to clean those tooth spaces.
You use a special string to fit in small places.
The Sugar Bugs come out with the string.
It's a very important thing we call flossing.

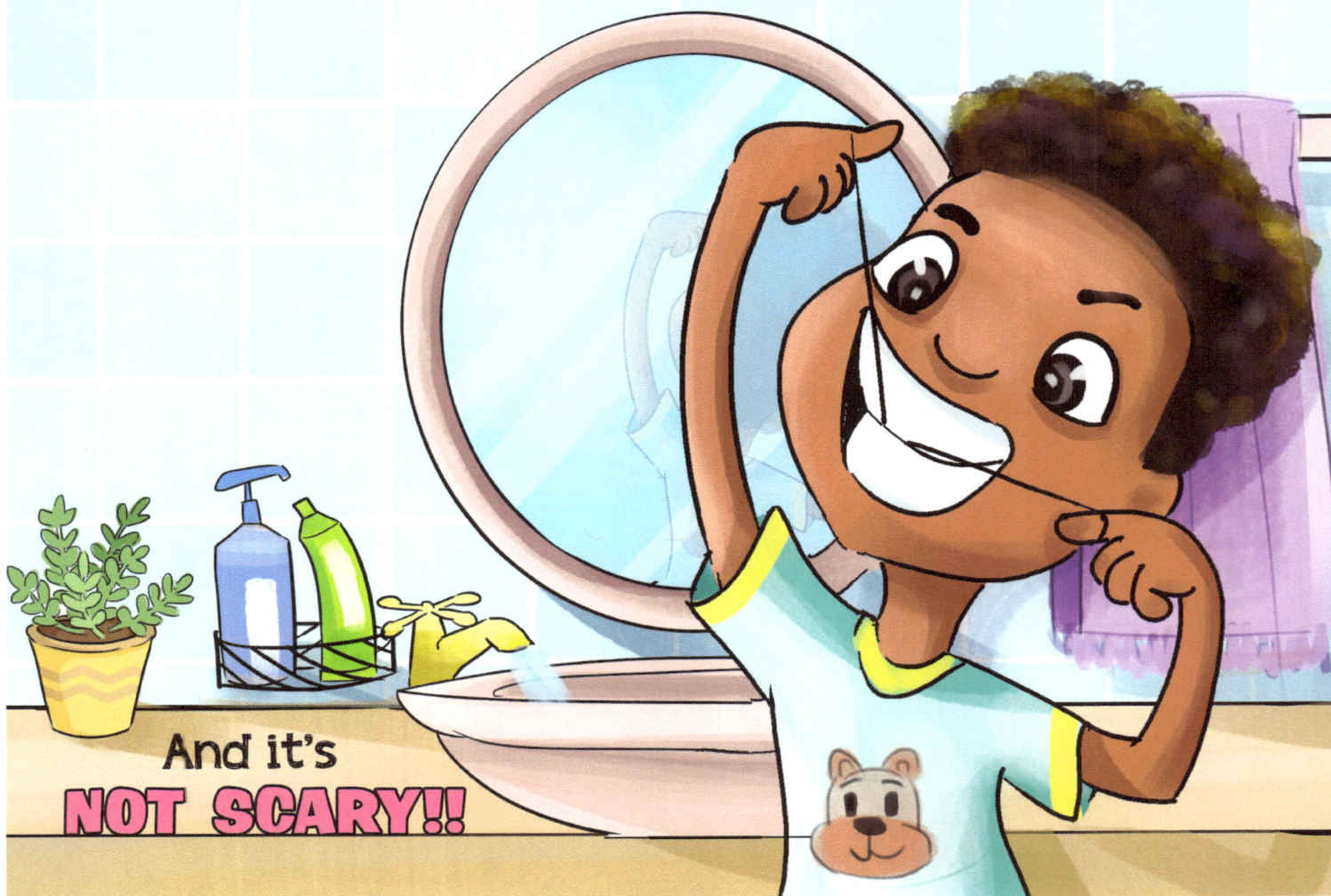

And it's
NOT SCARY!!

Your dental friends teach you about foods that are good for your chompers.

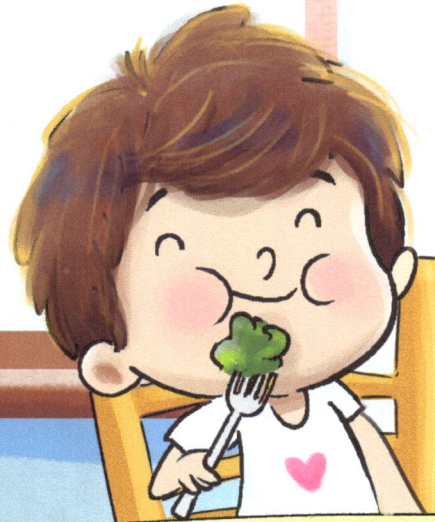

Milk or Almond Milk

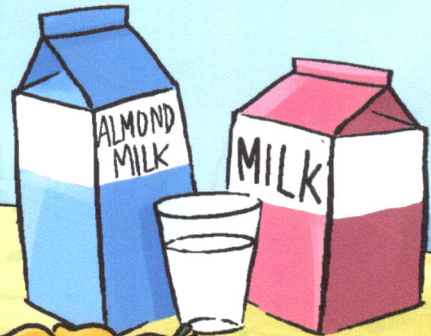

Peas and broccoli

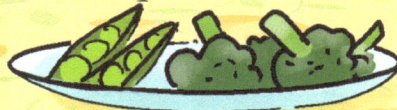

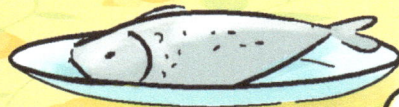

Eggs and Fish

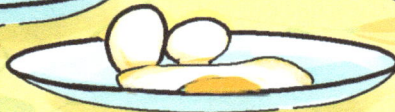

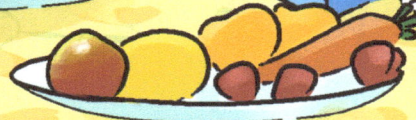

Oranges and Strawberries
Carrots and apples

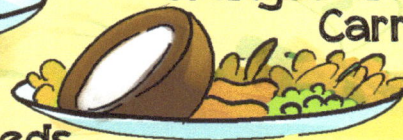

Nuts and Seeds

Foods like these are SUGAR BUG blockers.
Eating healthy is NOT SCARY!!

Now you're at the end of your visit!
You were brave and strong.
The dentist's office isn't scary at all, is it?
Come back again in 6 months and have some more fun.
Going to the dentist is great for everyone!

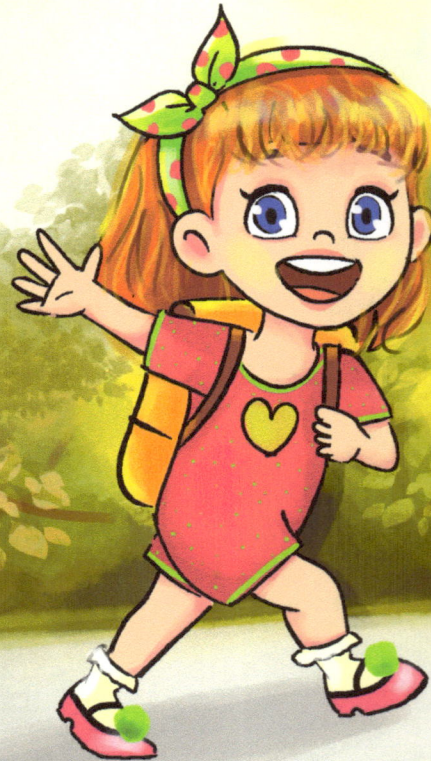

And it's (say it loud and proud!!)
NOT SCARY!!

Funny jokes to tell your dentist

1. Question: Which is the best day to go to the dentist?
Answer: Tooth-day.

2. Question: How far is it to the dentist's office?
Answer: Six smiles.

3. Question: What is a dentist's favorite dinosaur?
Answer: Floss-iraptor.

4. Question: Why did the iPhone go to the dentist?
Answer: She had bluetooth.

5. Question: What do dentists call their patients' X-rays?
Answer: Tooth pics.

6. Question: How do dentists brush their hair?
Answer: With a fine-toothed comb.

7. Question: What do you call a tooth that you lose in your backyard?
Answer: A lawn molar.

8. Question: Why did the jewel thief break into the dentist office?
Answer: He heard they had pearly whites.

9. Question: What do you call a bear that has no teeth?
Answer: A gummy bear.

10. Question: Why did the girl go back into the dentist's office while she was leaving?
Answer: Toothank him.

About the Author

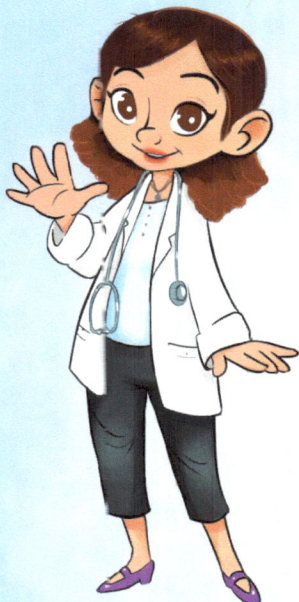

Tana Holmes is the author and creator of beautifully illustrated and creatively constructed books for children of all ages. She is best known for The History Tree Series, where the story-telling tree asks the young reader, "If old trees could talk, what tales could they tell?" The Old Patriarch Tree is set in Holmes' native Wyoming, in Grand Teton National Park. The Dueling Oak relates tales of New Orleans since its founding, and her best-known work, Alamo Tree has earned high praise from Texas historians, teachers, and parents alike. The unique use of easy reader combined with "Reader Guidance" footnotes helps the adult reader enrich the content as the child's development warrants. Holmes' new series, The NOT Scary Books, uses fantasy and familiar experiences to create tear-free, fear-free adventures out of first-time visits. The unknowns of the doctor, the dentist, daycare, and other dreaded outings have changed from fearful, to fascinating and fun.

Mrs. Holmes has a background in emergency medicine and public administration prior to choosing a career as a health science educator. Entering her 3rd decade of teaching medicine to high school and college students, she divides her time between teaching and authorship. Home is Houston, Texas with her firefighter husband and two rescue dogs. Her adult daughter and son in law are not far away in Austin.

If you enjoyed this book, please consider leaving a review. For more information about Tana Holmes and her books, please visit
www.tanaholmes.com, or follow her on
Twitter https://twitter.com/ TanaHolmesAuthr
Facebook https://www.facebook.com/ TanaHolmesAuthor
Instagram https://www.instagram.com/ tanaholmesauthor
Goodreads https://www.goodreads.com/author/show/19919054.Tana_S_Holmes
And Amazon https://www.amazon.com/~/e/B083RLLKV6

About the Illustrator

Mahfuja Selim is a freelance illustrator mostly working on children's books for 9 years. Her semi-cartoony drawing style sets her apart in the field. Her work has been published throughout the world in children's books, magazines, educational publications, children's games and packaging. She works with modern digital drawing tools at hand combined with all the traditional knowledge.
She spends most of her time with her lovely little daughter, Zoyee Mayamin. She enjoys fun activities with Zoyee, finding inspiration for the next illustration. Children love her work.

You can visit her portfolio here
Facebook https://www.facebook.com/amazingMahfuja
Instagram https://www.instagram.com/amazingmahfuja/
www.artstation.com/amazingmahfuja

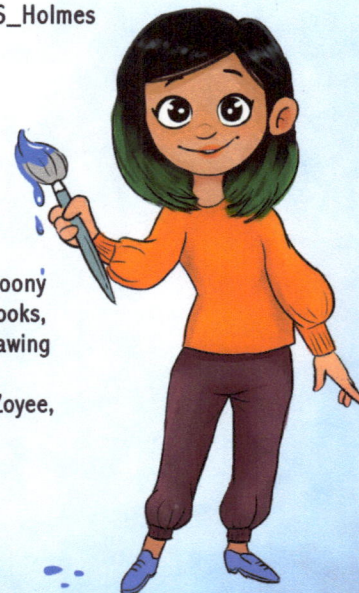

www.ingramcontent.com/pod-product-compliance
Lightning Source LLC
Chambersburg PA
CBHW061155030426
42336CB00003B/47